Hermeland Gomongo Tevolo

# Severe malaria in children aged 6 to 60 months

Hermeland Gomongo Tevolo

# Severe malaria in children aged 6 to 60 months

## Frequency of severe malaria in children aged 6 to 60 months at Kinkanda/Matadi Provincial Referral Hospital, DRC

ScienciaScripts

**Imprint**



Cover image: www.ingimage.com

This book is a translation from the original published under ISBN 978-3-330-87114-4.

Publisher:
Sciencia Scripts
is a trademark of
Dodo Books Indian Ocean Ltd. and OmniScriptum S.R.L publishing group

120 High Road, East Finchley, London, N2 9ED, United Kingdom
Str. Armeneasca 28/1, office 1, Chisinau MD-2012, Republic of Moldova, Europe
Managing Directors: Ieva Konstantinova, Victoria Ursu
info@omniscriptum.com

Printed at: see last page
**ISBN: 978-620-8-50840-1**

# *FREQUENCY OF SEVERE MALARIA IN CHILDREN AGED 6-60 MONTHS AT THE KINKANDA/MATADI PROVINCIAL REFERENCE HOSPITAL*

# INTRODUCTION

## 1. Background and justification for the study

Malaria is a febrile, haemolytic erythrocytopathy caused by the presence and development in the human body of one or more haematozoa of the genus Plasmodium, which are transmitted by the infesting bite of a mosquito (female Anopheles) of the Culicidae family (Karembe, 2013).

Because of its frequency and severity, malaria remains one of the most important public health problems in tropical countries today. Out of a world population of around 5.4 billion, 2.2 billion people are exposed to malaria infections in 90 countries.

The WHO estimates that there are 300-500 million cases of malaria in the world each year, over 90% of them in Africa. Mortality due to malaria is estimated at around 2 million per year (1 death every 30 seconds) and 90 percent (%) of these deaths occur in African children (SANOGO, 2021).

According to the World Malaria Report 2019, most cases of malaria (93%) were recorded in the African region in 2018, with 85% of malaria cases recorded in 19 sub-Saharan African countries and India. Six countries alone recorded more than half the cases: Nigeria (25%), DRC (12%), Uganda (4%), and Côte d'Ivoire, Mozambique and Niger (4% each) (WHO, 2019).

In Mali, malaria is the leading cause of morbidity in the general population and mortality in children under the age of 5. According to the statistical yearbook of the Local Health Information System (SLIS 2018), malaria is the leading reason for consultation with 32% of cases. According to the SLIS, in 2017, 2,439,995 cases of malaria were recorded, 32.44% of which occurred in children under 5 (SLIS, 2018). Malaria remains one of the most widespread and deadly parasitic diseases in the Democratic Republic of Congo (DRC), despite significant progress in the fight against this scourge. According to the WHO's World Malaria Report 2016, there has been a significant reduction in malaria cases from 28 million in 2010 to 19 million in 2015, and in malaria deaths from 82,000 in 2010 to 42,000 in 2015. According to the 2015 annual report produced by the DRC's National Malaria Control Programme (PNLP), 12,186,639 cases of malaria and 39,054 deaths attributed to this disease were recorded during that year (PNLP, 2017). We understand from what follows that despite the efforts made in the fight against malaria, this disease is still frequent and lethal for children under 6 to 60 months. This is the reason for our study of the current frequency of different forms of severe malaria in children aged 0 to 60 months in the Kinkanda Provincial Reference Hospital.

## 2. Objectives:

### 2.1. General :

- To determine the frequency of different forms of severe malaria in children in the paediatric ward of the HPRK.

### 2.2. Specific :

- To determine the hospital frequency of children aged 6-59 months admitted for severe malaria to the paediatric ward of the HPRK during the study period;
- Describe the socio-demographic characteristics of these children;
- To describe the clinical and biological characteristics of severe malaria in children aged 6-59 months at HPRK
- To determine the outcome of these children after care.

# CHAPTER I

# GENERAL INFORMATION

## 1. Definition

Malaria is a febrile, haemolytic erythrocytopathy caused by the presence and multiplication in the human body of a haematozoan of the genus Plasmodium. It is transmitted to humans by the infecting bite of a female mosquito of the genus Anopheles (Gentilini, 1993). Malaria is a febrile, haemolytic erythrocytopathy caused by the presence and multiplication in the blood of a haematozoan of the genus Plasmodium. It is transmitted to humans by the infecting bite of a mosquito of the genus Anopheles (KALOSSI, 2019).

## 2. Geographical breakdown

Malaria transmission is high in the inter-tropical zone. It is possible to draw up a broad outline of the geographical distribution of malaria throughout the world. It is also important to understand that because of the epidemiological factors influencing malaria transmission (distribution of Anopheles, vectorial capacity, biological characteristics of the different Plasmodium species), the geographical distribution varies from one continent to another, from one region to another, from one country to another and even from one village to another.

➢ **America**: North America is malaria-free. On the other hand, malaria exists in Central America (especially P.vivax), but the Caribbean islands are malaria-free, with the exception of Haiti. There is no transmission in the Lesser Antilles: Guadeloupe and Martinique. In South America, there are major outbreaks of P. falciparum (resistant to 4-amino-quinoleins) and P. vivax. Malaria is still rife in French Guyana, but mainly along rivers and in forests. Generally speaking, all

American cities are malaria-free except Amazonia.

- **Asia**: Malaria transmission is moderate in Asia Minor, the Indian peninsula, southern China, Thailand, Vietnam, Cambodia and Laos. Transmission in Asia takes the form of scattered outbreaks in rural, forested hilly areas. All major Asian cities are free of the disease except India.
- **Europe**: Malaria has been eradicated. Temporary reintroductions may occur and isolated cases may occur (airport malaria). But it is essentially imported malaria (travellers' malaria).
- **Oceania**: Transmission is heterogeneous. Some islands are affected (New Guinea, Solomon Islands, Vanuatu), while others are completely free: French Polynesia, New Caledonia, Wallis and Futuna, Fiji, Hawaii, etc. Australia and New Zealand are free of the disease.
- **Africa**: Malaria exists to a small extent in North Africa, where the species P. vivax and P. malariae are found. It is widespread throughout inter-tropical Africa, where P. falciparum, P. ovale and, to a lesser extent, P. malariae coexist. In some parts of Africa, P. vivax is also found. Generally, areas of high endemicity in Africa start in the Sahara sub-region and extend into the equatorial zone (A. TRAORE, 2019).

## 3. Etiopathogenesis

### 3.1. Pathogens

Malaria transmission is a complex process involving three organisms: the parasite (Plasmodium), the vertebrate host (Man) and the mosquito vector (Anopheles). The interaction between these three elements is largely influenced by the environment, with its biological, physical, climatic and human components.

### 3.1.1. The parasite

#### 3.1.1.1. Taxonomic definition

Malaria is caused by a protozoan parasite of the genus Plasmodium. Plasmodiums are intracellular (intraglobular) parasites that belong to the kingdom Animal, the sub-kingdom Protozoa, the phylum Api complexa, the class Sporozoae, the sub-class Coccidia, the order Eucoccidiida, the sub-order Haemosporiina, the family Plasmodiidae and the genus Plasmodium. There are 146 different species capable of infecting various hosts: Humans, monkeys, birds, rodents, reptiles, amphibians, bats, ungulates (antelope, etc.). 5 species are found in human blood: Plasmodium falicparum (Pf), Plasmodium vivax (Pv), Plasmodium ovale (Po), Plasmodium malariae (Pm) and plsamodium Knowlesi (WUMBA di Mosi NKOYI, 2017).

#### 3.1.1.2. Evolutionary cycle :

The cycle takes place successively in humans (asexual phase) and in anopheles (sexual phase).

➢ **In men, the cycle is divided into 2 phases:**

- **The hepatic or pre-erythrocytic or exo-erythrocytic phase:** this corresponds to the incubation phase, which is clinically asymptomatic.
- **The blood or erythrocyte phase:** this corresponds to the clinical phase of the disease.

**The exo-erythrocytic cycle:** this begins with the inoculation of the sporozoite (the stage that infects humans) when the mosquito bites. During a blood meal, the Plasmodium-infected Anopheles mosquito inoculates sporozoites into the human host.

#### 3.1.1.2.1. In men

##### 3.1.1.2.1.1. Pre-erythrocytic schizogony

Inoculated sporozoites remain in the skin, lymph and blood for up to thirty minutes. Many (around 90%) are destroyed within 60 minutes by the molecules of the reticuloendothelial system, particularly macrophages, but only less than 10% reach the hepatocytes. This sequestration of sporozoites occurs via the interaction of Circums porozoite protein (CSP), a major protein on the surface of sporozoites, and thrombospondin-related anonymous protein (TRAP), with the glycosaminoglycans (GAGs) prominent in the hepatic sinusoids. The sporozoites then cross the space of Disse and actively penetrate the hepatocytes by invagination of the plasma membrane, resulting in the formation of a parasitophorous vacuole. Sporozoites can also enter hepatocytes by membrane effraction without forming a vacuole, and migrate through several cells before finally infecting a hepatocyte by forming a vacuole. They differentiate into pre-erythrocytic schizonts (multinucleated form) which, after 2 to 7 days of maturation (formation of the blue body measuring between 35 and 50 μ in diameter), burst and release thousands of merozoites into the blood (10,000 to 40,000 merozoites depending on the species, which surround themselves with a particular cytoplasm (WUMBA di Mosi NKOYI, 2017). In the hepatocytes, the presence and multiplication of the parasite go unnoticed: the patient is in an incubation period. The hepatic cell parasitised by a schizont (from the sporozoite) becomes considerably enlarged (30 to 40 μm in diameter) and will be destroyed by the development of the parasite, but inflammatory phenomena remain discreet. Hepatic schizogonia is asymptomatic (WERY, 1995). The sporozoites enter the hepatocytes by sliding over the Kupffer cells and endothelial cells (this is referred to as a permissive role), but they do so through a type of fenestration known as the HSPG. On exiting to enter the sinusoidal circulation, these thousands of merozoites camouflage themselves opposite phagocytic Kupffer cells and epithelial cells by surrounding themselves with a membrane of the destroyed hepatocyte and will be called a mesosome (WUMBA di Mosi NKOYI, 2017). Maturation of these schizonts lasts one to two weeks and produces numerous (up to 2,000) merozoites, a parasitic stage that invades the bloodstream. Hepatic schizogony is unique in the cycle, as liver cells can only be infected by sporozoites. In P.vivax and P.Ovale infections, certain intrahepatic sporozoites remain quiescent (hypnozoites), and are responsible for a delayed hepatic schizogony leading to the release of merozoites into the blood several months after the mosquito bite, thus explaining the late relapses observed with these 2 species. Hypnozoites do not exist in P. falciparum infection (no relapse) and have not been demonstrated in P. malariae infection either, late relapses probably being due to the persistence of the parasite in the lymphatic ducts (WUMBA di Mosi NKOYI, 2017).

**3.1.1.2.1.2. Erythrocytic schizogony**

Merozoites penetrate red blood cells very rapidly (less than 60 minutes). Penetration of the merozoite into the erythrocyte and its maturation into a trophozoite (first young in the form of a "ring form") then into a mature schizont (rosette-shaped body) takes 48 or 72 hours (depending on the species) and leads to the destruction of the host red blood cell and the release of 8 to 32 new merozoites. These merozoites enter new red blood cells and begin a new cycle of replication. This part of the cycle corresponds to the clinical phase: the parasitaemia rises, the parasites progressively evolve at the same rate (they are said to become synchronous), all the erythrocyte schizonts mature at the same time, leading to the destruction of a large number of red blood cells periodically, every 48 hours (third fever of P. falciparum, P. vivax or P. ovale) or every 72 hours (fourth fever of P. malariae). In practice, it has been observed that third grade fever due to P. falciparum is rarely synchronous. Some merozoites undergo maturation in a red blood cell over around ten days, accompanied by sexual differentiation: they transform into male and female gametocytes

(WUMBA di Mosi NKOYI, 2017).

### 3.1.1.2.2. In female Anopheles

Gametocytes, ingested by the mosquito during a blood meal on an infected subject, are transformed into male gametes (8 microgametes by a metabolic process of ex flagellation) and a single female macrogamete (by disappearance of the chromatin corpuscle) which fuse after fertilisation and are transformed after 24 to 48 hours into a free, mobile egg called an ookinete. This ookinete, which measures around 10μ in length, must leave the digestive lumen and then attach itself between the outer wall of the stomach and the serosa, transforming into an oocyst measuring 50 to 80μ in diameter. Through a process of sporogenesis, these parasitic cells undergo differentiation (sporocysts, sporoblasts) leading to the formation of sporozoites which continue to multiply within this oocyst, producing hundreds of other sporozoites which initially spread throughout the mosquito's body but then migrate to the mosquito's salivary glands where they acquire their infective character. These sporozoites (which measure 11 to 14 μ in length and 0.5 to 1 μ in thickness) are the infective forms. ready to be inoculated with the mosquito's saliva during a blood meal on a vertebrate host (100 to 1000 sporozoites are injected at each meal in a vertebrate host (WUMBA di Mosi NKOYI, 2017).

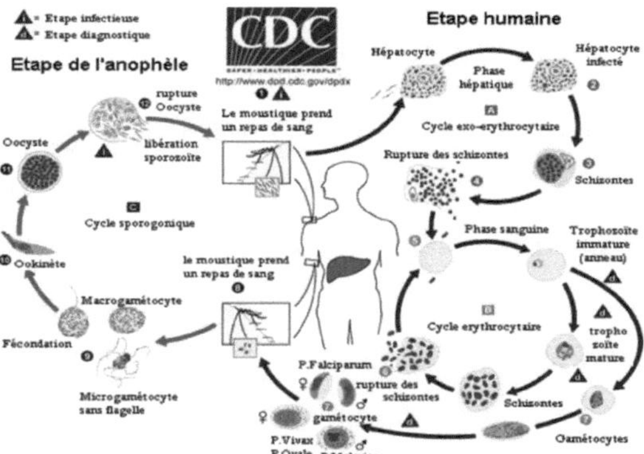


**Figure 1: Plasmodium cycle**

### 3.1.2. The vector

#### 3.1.2.1. Systematics

All primate Plasmodium, including the 5 species which parasitise humans, are transmitted by mosquitoes of the genus Anopheles (etymologically, from the Greek "a" privative and "Opheles" useful, in other words insect devoid of utility). Anopheles belong to the ^phylium of arthropods, to the class of insects, and to the ^phylium of insects. the order Diptera, the sub-order Nematicera, the family Culiciidae, the sub-family Anophelinae and the genus Anopheles. The Anopheles gebra comprises around 400 species, of which only around sixty are vectors of Plasmodium in natural conditions. Twenty species are responsible for most human cases (Mouchet & Camevale, 1991), Rodhain and Perez 1985).

## 4. Pathophysiology

The pathophysiology of malaria is still imperfectly understood, but the repercussions of malaria infection on certain organs have been well described.

### 4.1. The blood

The erythrocytic schizogony phase leads to haemolysis, which causes severe progressive anaemia in young children and pregnant women. The haemoglobin released by haemolysis causes renal overload and is partially converted to bilirubin in the liver. The excess is eliminated in the urine, resulting in haemoglobinuria. In addition, the parasite's use of haemoglobin leads to the precipitation in its cytoplasm of pigment granules (haemozoin), the release of which when the red blood cell bursts is partly responsible for the fever. The pigment, accumulated in the cytoplasm of the schizont, is released into the plasma when the merozoites are released. It is then phagocyted by monocyte-macrophages and neutrophil polynuclear cells (melaniferous leukocytes).

Platelets are sequestered by as yet poorly defined, probably immunological, mechanisms. The result is thrombocytopenia, biological disturbance frequently and early observed during a malaria attack(ANOFEL, 2014).

### 4.2. Spleen

The spleen is hypertrophic, soft and congestive. Its characteristic dark red, sometimes brown colour is due to the accumulation of pigment internalised by phagocytes. The increase in volume is caused by hypertrophy of the white pulp (lymphocytes, reticular cells, macrophages). Phagocytic activity involves parasitized red blood cells, cellular debris and parasite pigment. Histologically, during progressive visceral malaria, the spleen is huge, fibro-congestive and dark on section with lymphoid and histiocytic hyperplasia but parasites are rare in it (ANOFEL, 2014).

### 4.3. The liver

Exo-erythrocytic schizogony produces no inflammatory lesions. The destruction of a number of parenchymal cells by the schizonts goes unnoticed. There is hyperplasia of the Küpffer cells responsible for phagocytosis of cellular debris and haemozoin, associated with haemosiderin deposits. Pigment deposits subsequently invade the portal spaces within lympho-histiocytic infiltrates (ANOFEL, 2014).

### 4.4. Pathophysiology of severe seizures

Cerebral malaria and anaemia are the major complications of P. falciparum malaria. Initially based on post-mortem anatomopathological studies carried out on patients who had died of neuromalaria, a great deal of research has been carried out to elucidate its pathophysiology. Several theories, which are probably complementary, have now been put forward, including the sequestration of red blood cells parasitised by mature forms of Plasmodium, adhering to the endothelial cells of the microvessels, and the intervention of cytokines or other mediators(ANOFEL, 2014).

### 4.4.1. Sequestration

Aged forms of P. falciparum (aged trophozoites, schizonts) disappear from the peripheral bloodstream and are sequestered in the capillaries of deep organs (brain, kidneys, lungs, etc). This sequestration is due, at least in part, to cellular adhesion (cytoadherence) between the parasitized red blood cells and the endothelial cells of these capillaries. This cytoadherence is dependent on interactions between molecular receptors present on the surface of parasitized red blood cells (PfEMP1) and specific endothelial cell receptors (ICAM-1). This sequestration can also be accentuated by blockages in the capillaries due to reduced deformability of the parasitized red blood cells, and the formation of "rosettes": aggregates made up of a parasitized red blood cell to which several non-parasitized red blood cells adhere (ANOFEL, 2014).

### 4.4.2. Cytokines and other mediators

Pro-inflammatory cytokines (TNF-a, IFN-g, IL1, IL6, etc.) and various metabolic products (NO, lactic acid, etc.) are produced in a cascade during neuromalaria. Their action is probably combined with the circulatory blockage resulting from sequestration. Since experimental models are necessarily reductive, it is difficult to know how these different mechanisms work together in vivo. What has been described for the brain is probably also true for other organs (kidneys, lungs, placenta, etc.), explaining the multivisceral failure sometimes observed during a severe attack. It is now clear that the pathophysiology of severe malaria is probably much more complex than was initially thought (ANOFEL, 2014).

## 5. Diagnosis

### 5.1.Clinical manifestations

#### 5.1.1. Simple malaria

After a silent incubation phase, invasion of the erythrocytes is marked by a progressively rising fever reaching 39-40°C. The clinical picture is one of headache, myalgia and febrile gastric embarrassment (anorexia, abdominal pain, nausea and sometimes vomiting). The clinical picture is characterised by headaches, myalgias and febrile gastric discomfort (anorexia, abdominal pain, nausea and sometimes vomiting).During the primary invasion phase, malaria attacks are characterised by a succession of three stages, each with its own rhythm:

- **Shivering stage:** violent shivering with a sensation of intense cold and a fever of 39°C.
- **A heat stage:** no shivering, with a fever of 40-41°C.
- **A sweating stage**: profuse sweating and a temperature of 37°C.

The manifestations of malaria attacks vary according to the plasmodial species. They occur every 2 days when schizogony lasts 48 hours, giving rise to a third fever (P. vivax, P. ovale and P. falciparum), or every 3 days when schizogony lasts 72 hours, giving rise to a fourth fever (P. malariae) and a daily fever in the case of P. knowlesi. If left untreated or poorly treated, uncomplicated malaria can develop into severe malaria (A. TRAORE, 2019).

#### 5.1.2. Severe and complicated malaria

##### 5.1.2.1. Definition [26]

The definition of severe malaria given in 1990 by WARRELL D.A et al is the most widely accepted. According to these authors, severe malaria is defined as the presence of asexual haematozoa in the blood associated with one or more of the following signs:

**a. Neuromalaria:** deep coma reactive to nociceptive stimuli, excluding other causes of encephalopathy (hypoglycaemia, meningoencephalitis, eclampsia and metabolic comas).

**b. Severe anaemia** with a haematocrit level of <15% (haemoglobin level <5 grams (g) / decilitre (dl) in the absence of any other cause of anaemia.

**c. Renal failure** with urinary excretion <2 millitre (ml) / kilogram (kg) / 24 hours and serum creatinine >265 micromol/ litre (l) or 3 milligram (mg)/100 millilitres (ml).

**d. Pulmonary oedema or respiratory distress syndrome.**

**e. Hypoglycaemia** with blood glucose <2.2mmol/l or 0.4g/l.

**f. Circulatory collapse** manifested by systolic blood pressure <50mmHg in children aged 1 to 5 years or <70 millimetres of mercury (mmHg) in children aged over 5 years associated with cold, clammy skin or a central and peripheral temperature difference greater than 100°C.

**g. Diffuse spontaneous haemorrhage or Disseminated intravascular coagulation (DIC)**

**h. Spontaneous convulsions repeated more than twice in 24 hours despite cooling measures.**

**i. Acidaemia:** With an arterial pH <7.25 and **acidosis** with a plasma bicarbonate level <15 millimole (mmol)/l.

**j. Macroscopic haemoglobinuria.**

Apart from these major signs, there are minor criteria for severe malaria: a stage I coma, prostration or weakness with no other neurological cause.

Hyperparasitism with a parasite density of over 10% (500,000 trophozoites/microlitre of blood) (Mabiala-Babela, 2000).

Clinical jaundice or an increase in total bilirubin to 50 micromole/l. Major hyperthermia: ≥ 40°C.

**Table 1: Blantyre score**

| Types of response | Answer | Score |
|---|---|---|
| | Locating the painful stimulus | 2 |
| | Withdrawal of limb in response to pain | 1 |
| Best mortice response | Non-specific response or no response | 0 |
| | Appropriate crying | 2 |
| Best verbal response | Inappropriate whining or crying | 1 |
| | No | 0 |
| | Lead (follow mother's face) | 1 |
| Eye movements | Non-directed | 0 |
| Total Interpretation : | | 5 |

- Blantyre 0 = coma stage 4

- Blantyre 2 or 1 = stage 3 coma

- Blantyre 3 = stage 2 coma

- Blantyre 4 = coma stage 1

- Blantyre 5 = No coma

### 5.1.2.2. Clinical forms of severe malaria

#### 5.1.2.2.1. Cerebral malaria

**a. Onset**: may be gradual or abrupt.

A pernicious attack with a gradual onset is marked by the onset of irregular fever and a diffuse algesic syndrome, associated with digestive problems. Clinical examination may reveal a neurological component, suggesting the onset of severe malaria. Sudden-onset neuromalaria is characterised by a triad of symptoms (fever, coma, convulsions), frequently accompanied by respiratory distress. It is common in young children in endemic areas (< 5 years) and can lead to death within a few hours.

**b. State phase :**

The fever is usually very high and the neurological picture is complete and may include :

- **Disturbances of consciousness**: these are constant but of varying intensity, ranging from simple obnubilation to deep coma. The coma is generally calm, without neck rigidity (or very discreet), without photophobia, and accompanied by abolition of the corneal reflex.
- **Convulsions:** much more frequent in children than in adults,they may be inaugural. They may be generalised or localised, spaced out over time or, on the contrary, form a convulsive state. They can sometimes be pauci-symptomatic (clonic lips, facial muscles, rapid eye movements, excessive salivation). They must be distinguished from hyperthermic convulsions: to be recognised, they must be repeated over time ($\geq 2$ / 24 hours) with a post-critical phase of disturbed consciousness > 15 minutes.
- **Tonus disorders**: the patient is generally hypotonic. Stiffness and opisthotonos can be seen in very advanced forms and have a poor prognosis. Osteotendinous reflexes are variable, sometimes very sharp, exceptionally abolished (poor prognosis).
- **Other associated clinical signs**: neurological signs may predominate

They may also be associated with other visceral manifestations. Virtually any organ can be affected, including the kidneys, lungs (risk of pulmonary oedema) and liver. The picture is sometimes one of multiple visceral failure. Sometimes, without any obvious neurological signs, severe forms with profound anaemia are observed (in children).

**c. Terrain**: mainly non-immune individuals (children, women, pregnant women, new subjects) or after repeated simple attacks.

**d. Complications**: haemorrhage with DIC, acute renal failure, acute pulmonary oedema (APO), collapse, etc.

**e. Course**: If left untreated, the patient dies. With proper treatment, the disease may be cured with or without sequelae (hemiplegia, cortical blindness, cerebellar ataxia, severe hypotonia, mental retardation, behavioural problems, etc.) (ANOFEL, 2014).

**f. Poor prognostic factors**

- Pregnancy, splenectomy or other immunocompromised conditions
- Very high fever
- Hepatomegaly
- Parasitaemia >10
- Metabolic disturbances
- Hypoglycorrhachia and elevation of lactases Haematocrit <20%, haemoglobin <7g/dl
- Total bilirubin > 50 micrometres
- Oligoanuria with creatinemia >260 micrometres
- Respiratory distress (Pichard, 2002)

**5.1.2.2.2. Anaemia [28]**

It is the most common complication of P. falciparum malaria. It is due to the destruction of red blood cells, whether parasitised or not, and manifests itself clinically as :

- Very marked mucocutaneous pallor, often with frank or moderate jaundice.
- Confusion, asthenia, agitation, coma.
- Systolic murmur, gallop rhythm, tachycardia, heart failure.
- Polypnoea, chest indrawing, whining, nasal flaring.
- Hepatomegaly and/or splenomegaly (Pichard, 2002).

#### 5.1.2.2.3. Evolving visceral malaria

It is a chronic disease that affects mainly children living in endemic areas or adults who have not been immunised against the disease and who have been subjected to repeated parasitic inoculations. The clinical picture is characterised by severe anaemia (with pallor, dyspnoea, asthenia, anorganic murmurs and oedema), severe splenomegaly, fever of around 38°C, sometimes with more severe heat attacks and, in children, delayed growth and development. The parasite is found in the patient's peripheral blood (but the parasitaemia may be very low and the diagnosis difficult), malaria serology is positive but with a classically lower level of antibodies than in the presence of hyper-reactive malarial splenomegaly, the immunoglobulin G (IgG) level is high but the immunoglobulin M (IgM) level is normal. Progression under prolonged treatment is spectacular (M. TRAORE, 2007).

#### 5.1.2.2.4. Hyperreactive malarial splenomegaly (HMS)

Initially described as "Idiopathic Tropical Splenomegaly", HPS has mainly been described in natives living in malarious areas. Unlike progressive visceral malaria, it is more commonly seen in adults. It is a disease of immune complexes caused by an exaggerated reaction of the spleen to prolonged stimulation of mononuclear phagocytes by circulating immune complexes. The result is splenomegaly with hypersplenism. leading to a fall in the 3 blood lines and production of IgG and IgM in exaggerated quantities. Anti-malarial serology must be strongly positive in order to retain the diagnosis, which in the face of splenomegaly must remain a diagnosis of exclusion. Progression is favourable under antimalarial treatment, but very slow (M. TRAORE, 2007).

#### 5.1.2.2.5. Bilious haemoglobin fever

Now exceptional, it is not strictly speaking a manifestation of malaria, but merely a syndrome of immuno-allergic aetiology. Classically, it occurs in former P. falciparum malaria sufferers who have undergone chemoprophylaxis, often irregular, with quinine for several years. It consists of intravascular haemolysis. The onset is sudden, marked by severe low back pain and prostration. Fever, vomiting of food and then vomiting of stools occur. Haemolytic jaundice appears with anaemia, collapse, oliguria or oligo-anuria made up of "port urine". Typical triggers include a new dose of quinine or cold ("landing fever"), but similar symptoms have recently been observed with halofantrine and mefloquine. The prognosis depends on how quickly the anaemia is corrected and diuresis resumed before progression to renal failure (M. TRAORE, 2007).

**5.1.2.2.6. Hypoglycaemia**

It may be due to liver dysfunction, excessive glucose consumption by maturing parasites or treatment with quinine, which increases insulin secretion by the pancreas. Hypoglycaemia is harmful to the brain, manifesting itself as consciousness disorders, generalised convulsions, abnormal postures and coma (M. TRAORE, 2007).

**5.1.2.2.7. Renal insufficiency**

As a complication, it is due to hypotension following dehydration or shock and occurs more often in adults.

**5.1.2.2.8. Cardiovascular collapse**

These patients are admitted in a state of cardiovascular collapse with systolic blood pressure $<70$mmHg. Clinically, the skin becomes cold, pale and cyanotic. The pulse is thready and sometimes impenetrable.

**5.1.2.2.9. Spontaneous haemorrhage**

Some patients may have spontaneous bleeding from the gums, external digestive tract or skin, or prolonged bleeding from injection sites. This is a serious coagulation disorder associated with disseminated intravascular coagulation, which can be rapidly fatal (Warrell, 1990).

#### 5.1.2.2.10. Pulmonary oedema

It may appear several days after chemotherapy, just as the patient's general condition is improving. The first sign is an increase in ventilatory rate, which precedes the appearance of the other signs: the classic tide of crackling rales with frothy sputum, often tinged with blood. In addition to these signs, hypoxia can lead to convulsions and a deterioration in consciousness, and death can follow within a few hours (Nanema, 2004).

#### 5.1.2.2.11. Hyperpyrexia [31, 32]

High fever is a common sign of severe attacks of P. falciparum malaria. Fevers above 39.5°C are associated with an increased frequency of convulsions; fevers between 39.5°C and 42°C with delirium, and above that with coma.

Hyperthermia can cause serious neurological sequelae in pregnant women and can result in foetal distress **(Sall 2006, Rép du Mali 2015).**

#### 5.1.2.2.12. Dehydration and acid-base disorders

Patients with severe P. falciparum malaria often present with the following on admission:

- **Signs of hypovolaemia**: low jugular venous pressure, orthostatic hypotension and oliguria with high urine density.

- **Signs of dehydration**: Decreased peripheral circulation, deep breathing (acidosis type), dehydration skin fold, increased uraemia (>6.5mmol/l), thirst, loss of 3 to 4% of total body mass, signs of metabolic acidosis.

#### 5.1.2.2.13. Hyperparasitemia [32]

As a general rule, and particularly in non-immune individuals, high parasite densities and peripheral schizontaemia are associated with major severity. However, in areas where malaria is endemic, particularly immune children can tolerate surprisingly high parasitaemia levels (20 to 30%), which are often clinically silent (Rép du Mali, 2015).

#### 5.1.2.2.14. Splenic rupture in malaria

They are particularly common in patients with large malarial tropical splenomegaly, as seen in progressive visceral malaria and idiopathic tropical splenomegaly syndrome. These splenic ruptures are either spontaneous or caused by minimal trauma. The mechanism of rupture is either torsion of the pedicle or splenic infarction with subcapsular haematoma.

P. vivax is usually responsible, while P. malariae and P. falciparum are rarely involved. More recently, spontaneous ruptures have been observed in chemoresistant P. falciparum malaria. This may be explained by acute splenic congestion in a spleen previously weakened by prolonged malaria infection.

## 5.2. Biological diagnosis

**5.2.1. Morphological method:** the oldest methods, still used in the laboratory, are based on direct microscopic observation of the morphology of the various parasites in red blood cells.

**5.2.2. Thick blood drop (TG):** this is a technique for concentrating red blood cells, enabling a qualitative study of the plasmodium by direct observation under the microscope: this is the diagnosis of certainty. It is the technique of choice in epidemiological investigations.

**5.2.3. The thin smear (FM):** also a reference method, it, like the thick drop, reveals intraerythrocytic haematozoa but is not recommended for quantitative assessment of parasitaemia.

### 5.2.4. Immuno-chromatographic method

The principle behind these tests is the detection of Plasmodium-specific proteins (HRP-2 antigens or pLDH and aldolase enzymes) by chromatography on a solid support. Some of these tests can now be used to confirm a positive diagnosis (presence of Plasmodium) and to diagnose the species: P. falciparum and/or another species. These rapid tests, which are very easy to use and packaged individually, are very practical and have good sensitivity (especially for P. falciparum if they detect the HRP-2 antigen), but do not measure parasitaemia and, in some cases, remain positive for several days after the plasmodia have disappeared from the blood (Nanema, 2004).

### 5.2.5. Optimal-ITTM

In this test, the antigen considered is lactate dehydrogenase (LDH), an enzyme found in the parasite's glycolytic mechanism. It is produced by the sexual and asexual plasmodial forms. Each species has a specific LDH. This specificity is used in this test to differentiate P. falciparum from other species. ParasightFTM and CoreTMMalaria (Plasmodium falciparum) (Pf): exclusively for the detection of Plasmodium falciparum, these tests are based on the capture of the Histidine-Rich-Protein (HRP)-2, one of the three Histidine-Rich-Protein synthesised by red blood cells infected by this parasite. This water-soluble protein, expressed on the surface of the erythrocyte membrane by asexual forms and young gametocytes.

### 5.2.6. Molecular biology

Diagnosis can also be made using the Polymerase Chain Reaction (PCR) technique. This method also makes it possible to study the genetic fingerprint of this species, provided that molecular markers are available. Markers are single-copy genes in the haploid genome of the parasite that can be used to estimate the number of parasites circulating in the peripheral blood, provided they are sufficiently polymorphic.

Candidate genes for this purpose must be stable during the asexual phase of the parasite life cycle and have a single copy of the gene per haploid parasite genome. PCR with such markers is desirable for studying parasite population dynamics. PCR diagnosis generally uses multiple-copy gene markers; in most cases, these sequences must be conserved and able to discriminate between species.

**5.2.7. Haematological and biochemical parameters of severe malaria** The tests reveal the presence or absence of P. falciparum, whether or not associated with à a anaemia.We observed usually a thrombocytopenia (100,000 platelets/µL) and in some cases the platelet count may be extremely low (less than 20,000 platelets/µL). Hyperleukocytosis may be seen in some children during the most severe forms. Plasma or serum concentrations of urea, creatinine, albumin, bilirubin and liver and muscle enzymes may be found. The titres of these liver enzymes are lower than those seen in viral hepatitis. In severe forms, children frequently present with acidosis, a drop in plasma pH and bicarbonate concentrations. There may be hydroelectrolytic disorders (sodium, potassium, chlorine, calcium, phosphorus). Lactate levels in plasma and cerebrospinal fluid (CSF) are increased, particularly in hypoglycaemic patients.

## 6. Treatment of uncomplicated malaria

According to the report from the National Malaria Control Programme (PNLP), treatment is carried out using Artemisinin-based Combination Therapies (ACTs).

- **Artesunate**: 4mg/kg/day for 3 days
- **Amodiaquine**: 25mg/kg/day for 3 days (A. TRAORE, 2019)

**Table 2: Treatment regimen for uncomplicated malaria with Artesunate + Amodiaquine (AS + AQ)**

| Weight/age group | Presentation | Day 1 | Day 2 | Day 3 |
|---|---|---|---|---|
| 4.5-8kg (2 to 11 months) | 25 mg/67.5 mg Blister pack of 3 cps | 1 Cp | 1 Cp | 1 Cp |
| 9-17 kg (1-5 years) | 50 mg/135 mg Blister pack of 3 cps | 1 Cp | 1 Cp | 1 Cp |
| 18-35 kg (6-13 years) | 100 mg/270 mg Blister pack of 3 cps | 1 Cp | 1 Cp | 1 Cp |
| ≥36 kg (14 years and over) | 100 mg/270 mg Blister pack of 6 cps | 2 Cp | 2 Cp | 2 Cp |

**Table 3: Treatment regimen for uncomplicated malaria with Artemether-Lumefantrine. Dosage of the Artemether (20 mg) - Lumefantrine (120 mg) combination.**

| Weight/age group | Day 1 Morning / Evening | Day 2 Morning / Evening | Day 3 Morning / Evening |
|---|---|---|---|
| 5-14 kg (2 months to 3 years) | 1 Cp / 1 Cp | 1 Cp / 1 Cp | 1 Cp / 1 Cp |
| 15-24 kg (4-6 years) | 2 Cp / 2 Cp | 2 Cp / 2 Cp | 2 Cp / 2 Cp |
| 25-34 kg (7-10 years) | 3 Cp / 3 Cp | 3 Cp / 3 Cp | 3 Cp / 3 Cp |
| >34 kg and adults | 4 Cp / 4 Cp | 4 Cp / 4 Cp | 4 Cp / 4 Cp |

## 7. Management of severe and complicated malaria

### 7.1.Principle

Children presenting with cerebral malaria or other severe manifestations must be treated as a medical emergency. Once the urgent management of a child with severe malaria has been initiated, a certain amount of information must be sought:

➢ The patient's place of residence and recent movements, because of the existence of areas where P. falciparum strains are multi-drug resistant.

➢ Ask the parents or accompanying adults to specify any anti-malarial or other treatments that may have been administered, as well as any recent fluid intake or urine output. A quick initial examination will determine hydration status and detect any pulmonary oedema or other serious symptoms.

➢ After taking a blood sample for GE/FM, haematocrit (Hte), Hb, blood sugar, etc. biological tests, treatment is started immediately after parasitological confirmation.

➢ Therapeutic measures to be taken immediately include correcting any hypoglycaemia, treating convulsions and bringing down an excessively high temperature.

➢ Once first aid has been started, vital signs and fluid balance must be monitored. Particular attention should be paid to fluid overload or depletion, haematocrit, parasitemia, blood glucose and other parameters as necessary (Rép du Mali, 2015) .

## 7.2.Resources

Treating malaria still poses problems today. Several classes of product have successively emerged, each with its own advantages and disadvantages. However, the range of medicines remains narrow. This is because the discovery of new antimalarial drugs seems laborious. In children with severe malaria, antimalarial drugs must be administered parenterally (Chandenier & Danis, 2000).

### 7.2.1. Artesunate

#### 7.2.1.1. Dosage of Artesunate

Artesunate 2.4 mg/kg body weight administered intravenously (IV) or intramuscularly (IM) on admission (t = 0), then 12 h and 24 h later and, thereafter, once a day until the patient is able to take oral medication. Variability of pharmacokinetic parameters according to particular situations and populations: Effect of malaria (stage, severity): the comparative data available are few and sometimes conflicting. It appears that systemic exposure to AS and DHA is increased in the initial phase of the malaria attack compared with the convalescence phase, and in malaria sufferers compared with healthy subjects (reduced clearance).

- Paediatric population: the available data are insufficient to reach a conclusion on this point.

Treatment over 5 days by weight and age appear to be significant factors of variability in the volume of distribution of DHA. Weight-based dosing limits this variability, but paediatric studies are needed to clarify the role of age.

### 7.2.2. Artemether

Intramuscular dose and method of administration: the dose is 3.2mg/kg body weight in one injection on admission, followed by 1.6mg/kg in one injection per day for 4 days (Ref = Management of severe malaria WHO/2013).

### 7.2.3. Quinine

Recommended dosage: National Malaria Control Programme (PNLP) participant's manual. Quinine administered by intravenous infusion :

- Loading dose: 20 mg quinine salt/kg) on admission in adults and children.

**NB:** The loading dose is only administered if the patient has not taken quinine in the previous 24 hours or Mefloquine in the previous 7 days. If the patient has taken quinine in the previous 24 hours or Mefloquine in the previous 7 days, the maintenance dose is used.

- Maintenance dose :

Children : Dosage: 10 mg/kg of quinine hydrochloride salts (8.3mg base) diluted in 10ml/kg of 10% glucose serum (or 4.3% dextrose or 0.9% saline for diabetics).

Duration of infusion: 2 to 4 hours Interval between the start of infusions: 8 hours Switch to oral artemisinin-based combination therapy (ACT) as soon as the patient can swallow.

## 7.3. Prevention

There are two methods of prevention: chemoprevention (pregnant women and children aged between 3 and 59 months) and vector control (WHO, 2014).

# CHAPTER II

# MATERIALS AND METHOD

## 2 .1. Type of study

This was a retrospective descriptive study. We adopted a non-probabilistic method with exhaustive and systematic recruitment of all cases of children admitted with severe malaria to the paediatric ward who met the inclusion criteria.

## 2.2. Study period

The study period ran from January 2022 to December 2023.

## 2.3. Presentation of the environment

The study was carried out in the town of Matadi, capital of the province of KC in the DRC, 352 km west of Kinshasa, and more specifically in the Kinkanda Provincial Reference Hospital. In 2023, Matadi's population was estimated at 431,505, with a surface area of 110 km². In terms of health, the city of Matadi is divided into two health zones (the Matadi health zone, divided into 12 health areas, and the Nzanza health zone, divided into 10 health areas). The Kinkanda provincial referral hospital is geographically located in the south-western part of the town of Matadi in the urban-rural commune of Matadi in the Matadi health zone and Hygiene B health area, on the road leading to the Republic of Angola via the municipality of Noqui. It is bounded:

- To the north, the small market of Kinkanda, the Sacré-Coeur Catholic Church, the building of the provincial health division and the provincial reference maternity hospital of Central Kongo;
- To the south by the Matadi health zone office and the neighbouring houses of ISIPA Matadi;
- To the east by the neighbouring dwellings of the Flat hôtel Ledya ;

➢ To the west by the control tower building and the dwellings adjacent to the Kinkanda mortuary.

The Kinkanda provincial referral hospital has 6 departments:

➢ Internal Medicine

➢ Emergency

➢ Paediatrics

➢ Gynaecology and obstetrics

➢ Surgery

➢ The Department of Screening, Prevention and Control of infectious diseases

The HPRK has a capacity of 246 beds (actual capacity) with an estimated capacity of 300 beds. It has more than 50 doctors, over 300 nurses and many paramedical professionals.

**2.4.Study population**

All children aged between 6 months and 5 years admitted to the paediatric ward for severe malaria were included in our study. 200 cases were retained after investigation during our study period. Files that could not be used, files of any child who died in the community and whose death was noted on admission, and cases of death from unknown causes were not included in our study.

**2.5.Sampling**

This is a non-exhaustive sample of all available medical records of children followed in the paediatric department of the HPRK during the period January 2022 to December 2023.

**2.5.1. Inclusion criteria**

➢ 6 months to 5 years old

➢ Have been diagnosed with severe malaria

- Have a complete file

### 2.5.2. Non-inclusion criteria

ALL folders that do not contain the parameters of interest.

## 2.6 Parameters of interest and operational definitions

### 2.6.1. Socio-demographic parameters

- Age
- Gender
- Weight

### 2.6.2. Clinical and biological values for severe malaria

- Fever, convulsions, coma, pallor, respiratory distress...
- GE

### 2.6.3. Operational definitions

- **Severe anaemia:** this is severe anaemia with an Hb level of less than 5g% or an Hct level of less than 15%.
- **Severe respiratory malaria:** respiratory distress, breathing difficulties associated with acidosis (PH less than 7.25) or hyper-lactatemia greater than 5mmol/l.
- **Neuromalaria:** profound and lasting impairment of consciousness (less than 6 hours, Blantyre score less than 2) without other obvious causes and neurological damage associated with the presence of an asexual form of the parasite.
- **Coma** is an abolition of consciousness and vigilance in response to stimulation with a Blantyre of less than 2.
- **Anemia** Hb level below 5g%.

## 2.7. Study tools

The tools used to develop this work are :

- The registers
- Patient records
- Collection sheets

## 2.8. Source, Organisation and Data Processing

We carried out a literature review using a survey form with an exhaustive examination of the files of all cases of severe malaria meeting our inclusion criteria.Once data collection was complete, it was organised, entered, encoded and stored in a database using Microsoft Office Excel 2016. The following variables were included: age, sex, weight, fever, convulsions, coma, pallor, respiratory distress, GE, etc.

Finally, the data was analysed using Excel 2016 software to produce the results.

## 2.9. Ethical considerations

The data was collected and processed in compliance with confidentiality rules.

## 2.10. Study limits

a. Health information problems

- Reporting bias
- Problems archiving patient files
- Poor completeness, promptness and accuracy of data collected
- Poor dissemination of quality information.

b. Descriptive and limited study at the Matadi Provincial Referral Hospital.

# CHAPTER III

# RESULTS

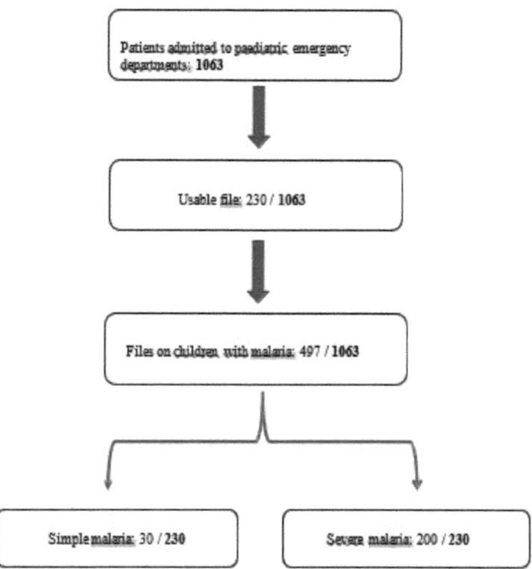


**Figure 2: Flow chart of children admitted to paediatric emergency departments**

## 1. Description of the characteristics of DM in the Matadi AS.

### a. Socio-demographic characteristics

#### ➢ Age groups

The highest proportion of children with malaria was in the 6-12 months age group (34%).

| Age group (Months) | Number of cases (n) | Proportion (%) |
|---|---|---|
| 6 - 12 | 68 | 34 |
| 13 - 24 | 56 | 28 |
| 25 - 36 | 39 | 19,5 |
| 37 - 48 | 17 | 8,5 |
| 49 - 60 | 20 | 10 |
| Total | 200 | 100 |

**Table 4: Breakdown of severe malaria cases by age**

- **Sex**

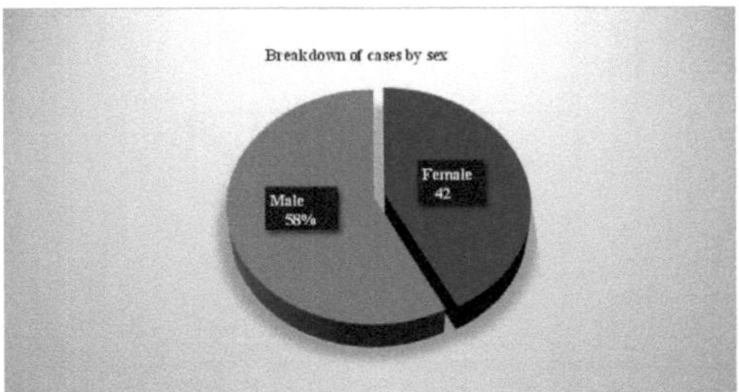


**Figure 3: Breakdown of severe malaria cases by sex**

The highest proportion of children admitted for severe malaria was among males (58%)

**b. Clinical and biological characteristics of malaria**

- **The shape**

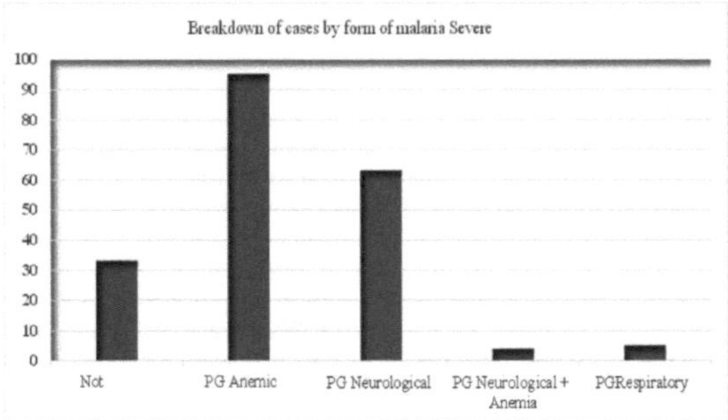


**Figure 4: Breakdown of severe malaria cases by form of malaria**

Severe anaemic malaria was the most common form with 47.5%, followed by severe neurological malaria (neuromalaria) with 31.5%.

> **Clinical signs**

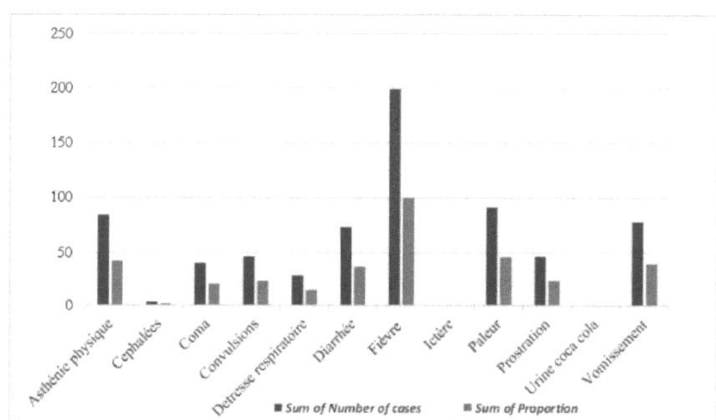


**Figure 5: Distribution of severe malaria cases by clinic**

The highest proportion of children admitted for severe malaria presented with fever (99.5%), pallor (45.5%), anaemia, physical asthenia (42%), vomiting (39%), diarrhoea (36.5%), convulsions (23%), prostration (23%), coma, etc. (20%), respiratory distress (14%), headaches (1.5%).

> **The number of trophos**

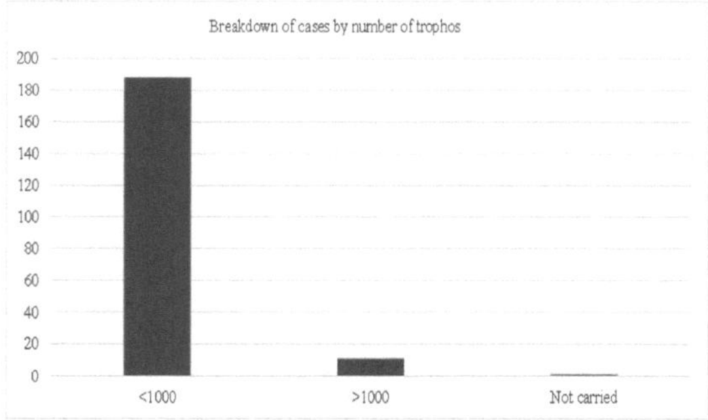


**Figure 6: Distribution of severe malaria cases according to the result of the thick blood smear test**

The highest proportion of children admitted for severe malaria was observed among those with fewer than 1,000 trophos, i.e. 94%.

## ➢ Care

Artesunate injection was administered to almost all children with severe malaria (98.5%) and 65.5% of these patients benefited from an ACT relay. Antibiotics (100%), blood transfusion (49%), anticonvulsants (26.5%) and oxygen therapy (13%) were the associated treatments for these patients.

**Table 5: Breakdown of severe malaria cases by type of management**

| PEC Malaria | Number of cases (n) | Proportion (%) |
|---|---|---|
| Artesunate | 197 | 98,5 |
| Quinine | 3 | 1,5 |
| ACT<br>Associated treatments | 131 | 65,5 |
| Antibiotics<br>Anticonvulsants<br>Transfusions<br>Oxygen therapy | 200<br>53<br>98<br>26 | 100<br>26,5<br>49<br>13 |

## ➢ Length of hospital stay

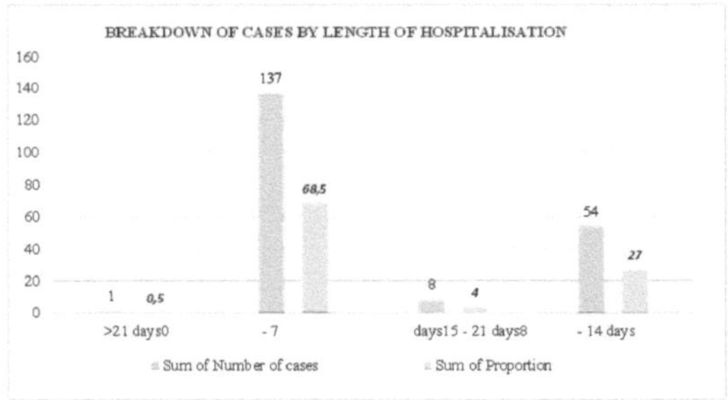


**Figure 7: Breakdown of severe malaria cases by length of stay in hospital**

The length of hospitalisation for children admitted with severe malaria varied between 0 and 7 days, representing a proportion of 68.5%.

## ➢ The evolution

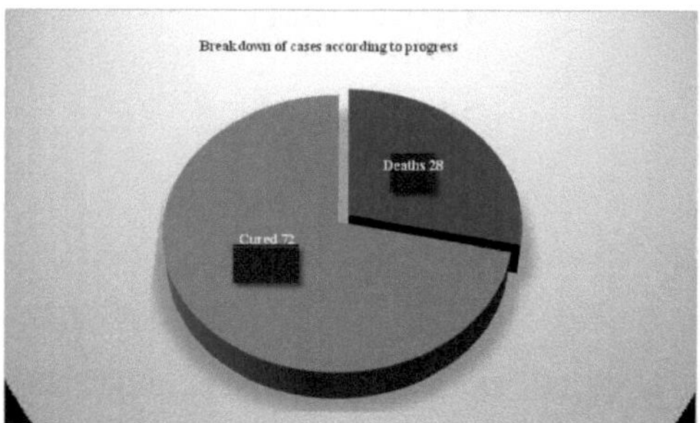


**Figure 8: Breakdown of severe malaria cases by course of illness**

72% of children admitted for severe malaria were cured.

# CHAPTER IV

# DISCUSSION

The aim of this study was to describe the frequency of different forms of severe malaria in children under 5 during the period 2022-2023 at the Kinkanda Provincial Referral Hospital. During our study period, the general paediatrics department hospitalised 1,063 children, 200 of whom had severe malaria, i.e. a prevalence of 18.8%. This prevalence is higher than that reported in 2018 at the Panda Hospital in Likasi, which found 221 patients with severe malaria out of 1653 children hospitalised, i.e. 13.4% of the total hospital population (Mutombo, Kamona, et al., 2018). In our study, we found a greater predominance of males, who accounted for 58% of cases, with a sex ratio of 1.35. Our results are comparable to those found in the literature, which show a predominance of males without any explanation (BOBOSSI-SERENGBE et al., 2006; Mutombo, Mukuku, et al., 2018; Sawadogo et al., 2024). Our results are superior to those reported by Mutombo, Kamona, et al. which show a 51.6% male predominance and a sex ratio of 1.06. The age groups most affected are those between 6 and 12 months. This can be explained by the fact that in holoendemic zones, protection before 6 months of age is ensured by a high haemoglobin F level and by antibodies passively transmitted by the mother, which gradually disappear, whereas after 5 years of age, active immunity prevents severe attacks (Mutombo, Kamona, et al., 2018). Our results contradict those of Mutombo, Kamona et al, Bobossi-Serengbe et al, and Koko, who reported a peak between 1 and 3 years of age (BOBOSSI-SERENGBE et al., 2006; KOKO et al., 1999; Mutombo, Kamona, et al., 2018). Clinically, fever was observed in 99.5% of patients. These results are consistent with the literature showing that fever is the primary reason for consultation for severe malaria. These results are similar to those found in the Central African Republic by **Serengbe G** et **al**, who noted in their studies that the main reason for consultation was fever. The main reason for consultation was fever (96.8%) (Bobossi Serengbe et al., 2004). These results contradict Rabenjarison et al. who found that, clinically, fever was observed in 5% of patients. In our study, the reasons for hospitalisation were dominated by anaemia (45.5%) followed by convulsions (23%). These results are similar to those of Traoré, in whom the reasons for hospitalisation were also dominated by anaemia (47.9%) followed by repeated convulsions (34.2%) (A. TRAORE, 2019).we believe that this would explain the clinical signs of severe malaria according to the literature. These results contradict Rabenjarison et al. on the clinical level, had a predominance of neurological signs such as disorder of consciousness (100%), obnubilation (17%), confusion (14%), and convulsion (11%)(RABENJARISON et al., 2018). In our study, the two main forms of severity were anaemia (47.5%) and neuromalaria (31.5%). These results are lower than those of Mutombo et al. who found a predominance of the anaemic form at 58.4% and cases followed by neuromalaria with a frequency of 46.2% (Mutombo, Kamona, et al., 2018). This would explain why Anaemia results from acute lysis of parasitized and non-parasitized red blood cells through rosettes and sequestration of red blood cells in the deep capillaries associated with medullary dyserythropoiesis during the first few days and explains the low reticulocytosis seen in malaria. Auto-agglutination of parasitised red blood cells: infected erythrocytes agglutinate and form micro-aggregates that can obstruct deep capillaries. Rosetting: aged parasitic red blood cells have knobbly protuberances which adhere to each other and to non-parasitised red blood cells, forming rosettes. Cyto-adhesion of parasitized red blood cells to vascular endothelium or placental trophoblastic cells enables Plasmodium to develop more easily thanks to a favourable gaseous environment (Haidaro et al., 1991). Self-medication, Longer delays in seeking care and inadequate treatment of uncomplicated malaria lead to severe malaria. Unlike Okoko, who divided the cases into 112 neurological forms and 101 anaemic forms (Okoko et al., 2016). In hospital, the specific antimalarial attack treatment is Artesunate-based (98.5%). Artesunate is the first-line treatment for severe malaria, as shown by our study and recommended by the WHO and the national malaria control programme. This is explained by the fact that intravenous Artesunate (compared with intravenous quinine) significantly reduced mortality in severe malaria, while being better tolerated and easier to use. In contrast, Mutombo et al. found that 90.5% of severe malaria cases were treated with infused or combined quinine salts (Mutombo, Kamona, et al., 2018). Our study showed an average length of hospitalisation of 7 days, unlike Dembélé et al. who also found an average length of hospitalisation of 3 days (Dembélé et al., 2020). The longer duration of hospitalisation in our study compared with others is explained by the fact that our study site is a provincial hospital receiving complex cases of severe malaria. We recorded 72% recovery without sequelae, which is lower than the study carried out by Dembelé et al. in MALI, which showed 82.9% recovery without sequelae, and Mutombo et al. is slightly lower than our study, with a recovery rate of 64.7% (Dembélé et al., 2020; Mutombo, Kamona, et al., 2018). The mortality rate for severe malaria in this study was 28%. These results are lower than Mutombo et al. which was 35.3% with a difference of 7.3% (Mutombo, Kamona, et al., 2018). The high mortality rate is justified by the limits of our resuscitation resources and the delay in consultation. Delays in consultation are an African prerogative.

# CONCLUSION

At the end of our study, we found that there were two main forms of malaria severity. These were anaemia and neuromalaria. The figures for the mortality rate from severe malaria in the under-5s in this study show that malaria is still a public health problem, despite the many efforts that have been made, and highlight the scale of the problem, as well as its preventable nature, which calls for action on the part of all those involved, to better adapt strategies to the local context in order to prevent avoidable deaths now and in the future.

# OUTLOOK

With a view to future studies, the results of this work argue in favour of :

a) Operational outlook

- Awareness, availability and correct use of LLINs in our households
- Raising women's awareness of the need to consult a health facility as soon as the first symptoms of malaria appear in a child
- Regular refresher courses for healthcare staff on standards and guidelines relating to the fight against malaria.
- Improving the quality of, and access to, prenatal, perinatal and postnatal care to ensure safer motherhood.
- Strengthening the technical platforms of referral health facilities.
- Making the most of health information in our health systems.

b) The scientific outlook

- Carrying out in-depth studies into the factors explaining deaths from severe malaria at the HPRK and in the town of Matadi.

## REFERENCES BIBLIOGRAPHIQUES

1. ANOFEL. (2014). MALARIA.

2. Bobossi Serengbe, G., Ndoyo, J., Gaudeuille, A., Longo, J. D. D., Bezzo, M. E., Ouilibona, S. F., & Ayivi, B. (2004). Current aspects of severe childhood malaria in Central African paediatric hospitals. Médecine et Maladies Infectieuses, 34(2), 86- 91. https://doi.org/10.1016/j.medmal.2003.09.003

3. BOBOSSI-SERENGBE, G., NDOYO, J., MUKESHIMANA, T., FIOBOY, R., & AYIVI, B. (2006, April). Le paludisme grave de l'enfant à l'hôpital préfectoral of Bouar (Central African Republic). https://www.santetropicale.com/sites_pays/resume_oa.asp?id_article=673&revue=man&rep=rca

4. Chandenier, J., & Danis, M. (2000). Le traitement du paludisme : Actualité et perspectives.

5. Dembélé, A., Cissé, M., Diakité, A., Maïga, B., Doumbia, A., Dembélé, M., Coulibaly, O., Togo, P., Sacko, K., Konaté, D., Diall, H., Ahamadou, I., Sylla, M., Dicko, F., Sidibé, L., Togo, B., Coulibaly, Y., Diakité, F., & Koné, Y. (2020). Epidemio-clinical study of paediatric emergency referrals at C.H.U Gabriel Touré. MALI SANTE PUBLIQUE 2020, 10(2), 29- 33.

6. Gentilini, M. (1993). Tropical Medicine (5th edition). Flammarion.

7. Haidaro, S. A., Doumbo, O., Traore, A. H., Koita, O., Dembele, M., Dolo, A., Pichard, E., & Diallo, A. N. (1991). (Results of a one-year systematic study). Médecine d'Afrique Noire.

8. KALOSSI, I. (2019). Incidence of malaria in a cohort in a context of chemoprevention of seasonal malaria (CPS) in Kalifabougou (Kati). UNIVERSITÉ DES SCIENCES, DES TECHNIQUES ET DES TECHNOLOGIES DE BAMAKO.

9. Karembe, C. (2013). Frequency and lethality of severe and complicated malaria in the paediatric ward of Sikasso hospital.

10. KOKO, J., DUFILLOT, D., ZIMA-EBEYARD, A. M., DUONG, T. H., GAHOUMA, D., & KOMBILA, M. (1999). Aspects Cliniques et Approche Epidemiologique Du Paludisme De L'Enfant a Libreville, Gabon. Medecine d'afrique, 46. https://www.academia.edu/76843763/Aspects_Cliniques_et_Approche_Epidemiological_of_Child_Malaria_in_Libreville_Gabon

11. Mabiala-Babela, J. (2000). Management of malaria in children in Brazzaville hospitals.

12. Mouchet, J., & Camevale, P. (1991). Vectors and transmission, in Paludisme.

13. Mutombo, A. M., Kamona, Y. M., Tshibanda, C. N., Mukuku, O., Ngwej, D. T., Wembonyama, S. O., Luboya, O. N., & Lutumba, P. (2018). Severe malaria in children under 5 years of age at Panda Hospital in Likasi, Democratic Republic of Congo. Revue de l'Infirmier Congolais, 2, 4- 10.

14. Mutombo, A. M., Mukuku, O., Tshibanda, K. N., Swana, E. K., Mukomena, E., Ngwej, D. T., Luboya, O. N., Kakoma, J.-B., Wembonyama, S. O., Van Geertruyden, J.-P., & Lutumba, P. (2018). Severe malaria and death risk factors among children under 5 years at Jason Sendwe Hospital in Democratic Republic of Congo. Pan African Medical Journal, 29. https://doi.org/10.11604/pamj.2018.29.184.15235

15. Nanema, F. (2004). Epidemiological, clinical and biological study of childhood malaria in rural Sahelian areas of Burkina Faso.

16. Okoko, A. R., Angouma Oya, S. M., Moyen, E., Kambourou, J., Ekouya-Bowassa, G., Atanda, H. L., & Moyen, G. (2016). Severe malaria in children at the Centre Hospitalier et Universitaire de Brazzaville. Journal de Pédiatrie and de Puériculture, 29(6), 304- 309. https://doi.org/10.1016/j.jpp.2016.09.004

17. WHO. (2014, April). WHO progress report on the annual United Nations resolution on malaria.

18. WHO. (2019). The World Malaria Report 2019 at a glance.

https://www.who.int/fr/news-room/feature-stories/detail/world-malaria- report-2019

19. Pichard, E. (2002). Manual of infectious diseases by Africa (John Libbey eurotext).

20. PNLP. (2017). Rapport d' activités 2016. MInistère de santé publique, 9.

21. RABENJARISON, F., VELOMORA, A., RAMAROLAHY, A. R. N., & RAVELOSON, N. E. (2018). Clinical and therapeutic aspects of severe malaria in the Medical Intensive Care Unit of the Joseph Raseta University Hospital of Befelatanana, Antananarivo. JOURNAL OF ANAESTHESIA RESUSCITATION, EMERGENCY MEDICINE AND TOXICOLOGY, 10(2), 7- 9.

22. Republic of Mali (2015). Report of the survey on the verification of the use final of malaria control products in Mali 21 August to 17 September 2015. 33.

23. Rodhain, F., & Perez, C. (1985). Precis d'entomologie médicale et vétérinaire.

24. Sall, A. (2006). Incidence and management of severe and complicated malaria in the paediatric department of the CHU Gabriel Touré. UNIVERSITÉ DES SCIENCES, DES TECHNIQUES ET DES TECHNOLOGIES DE BAMAKO.

25. SANOGO, A. L. (2021). MORBIDITY AND MORTALITY OF SEVERE MALARIA IN CHILDREN AGED 6 TO 59 MONTHS IN THE PAEDIATRICS DEPARTMENT OF THE CSRÉF OF SIKASSO. UNIVERSITÉ DES SCIENCES, DES TECHNIQUES ET DES TECHNOLOGIES DE BAMAKO.

26. Sawadogo, A., Semde, A., Ouattara, S., Bonzi, Y., Lengani, H., Diallo, F., Dah, J., Kyelem, G., & Coulibaly, G. (2024, July). Clinical and developmental profile of haemodialysis chronic of Bobo Dioulasso. https://www.santetropicale.com/sites_pays/resume_oa.asp?revue=man&id_ar

ticle=3761&rep=burkina

27. SLIS. (2018, April 27). 2018 SYSTEM STATISTICAL YEARBOOK LOCAL HEALTH INFORMATION SYSTEM IN MALI. Ministry of Health and Hygiène Publique. http://www.sante.gov.ml/docs/AnnuaireSLIS2018VF du 27avril. pdf.

28. TRAORE, A. (2019). Epidemiological study of malaria in 2019 in a cohort of volunteers in Kalifabougo. UNIVERSITÉ DES SCIENCES, DES TECHNIQUES ET DES TECHNOLOGIES DE BAMAKO.

29. TRAORE, M. (2007). Evaluation of the morbidity and mortality of severe malaria in the paediatric ward of the CHU Gabriel Touré.

30. Warrell, D. A. (1990). Severe and complicated malaria (2nd Ed. Trans R Soc Trop Med And hyg, p. 84).

31. WERY, M. (1995). PROTOZOOLOGIE MEDICALE (UNIVERSITÉ DE BOECK). Agence francophone pour l'enseignement et la recherche.

32. WUMBA di Mosi NKOYI, R. (2017). PARASITOLOGY COURSE NOTES.

33. Koko J, Dufillot D, Zima-Ebeyard AM, Duong TH, Gahouma D, Kombila M. Clinical aspects and epidemiological approach to childhood malaria in Libreville, Gabon. Med Afr Noire 1999; 46 (1): 10-14.(12)

34. Mutombo MA, Mukuku O, Kabuya MS, Lubala T, Bugeme M, Ilunga PM, Mubinda KP, Mutombo KA, Luboya NO. Severe malaria and severe malnutrition in children aged 6-59 months. Rev. Méd. Gd. Lacs 2013; 2 (3): 416-424.

35. Savadogo M, Boushab MB, Kyélem N. Management of severe malaria in children under five years of age in peripheral health facilities in Burkina Faso. Méd Afr Noire 2014; 61 (3): 164-168.

36. Asse KV, Brouh Y, Plo KJ. Severe malaria in children at the Bouaké university hospital (CHU) in the Republic of Côte d'Ivoire. Archives de pédiatrie

2003; 10 (1): 62.

37. Imbert P, Gendrel D. Treatment of malaria in children: severe malaria. Med Trop 2002; 62: 657-664.

38. Mulumba MP, Muhindo MH, Motuta AC, Zanga MM, Akele C. A look at the treatment of severe malarial anaemia in a paediatric hospital in Kinshasa. Ann Afr Med 2008; 2 (1): 15-23.

39. Idro R, Jenkins NE, Newton CR. Pathogenesis, clinical features and neurological outcome of cerebral malaria. Lancet Neurol 2005;4(12):827-40. DOI : 10.1016/S1474-4422(05)70247-7.

40. Gay F, Zougbédé S, N'Dilimabaka N, Rebollo A, Mazier D, Moreno A. Cerebral malaria: what is known and what is on research. Rev Neurol 2012 ;168(3) :239-56. DOI(Dembélé et al., 2020).

41. Rasti N, Wahlgren M, Chen Q. Molecular aspects of malaria pathogenesis. FEMS Immunol Med Microbiol 2004 ;41(1) :9-26. DOI : 10.1016/j.femsim.2004.01.010.

42. Argy N, Houzé S. Severe malaria: from pathophysiology to novel therapeutics. Journal des Anti-infectieux 2014;16:13-17.

# TABLE OF CONTENTS

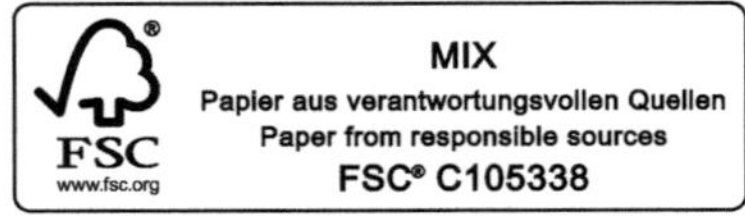


Printed by Books on Demand GmbH, Norderstedt / Germany